Teach Children About Nutrition

The Most Common Nutrition Myths and Real Nutritional Needs for Children

Frank Dixon

from various sources. Please consult a licensed professional before attempting any techniques outlined in this book.

Before we begin, I have something special waiting for you. An action-packed 1 page printout with a few quick & easy tips taken from this book that you can start using today to become a better parent right now!

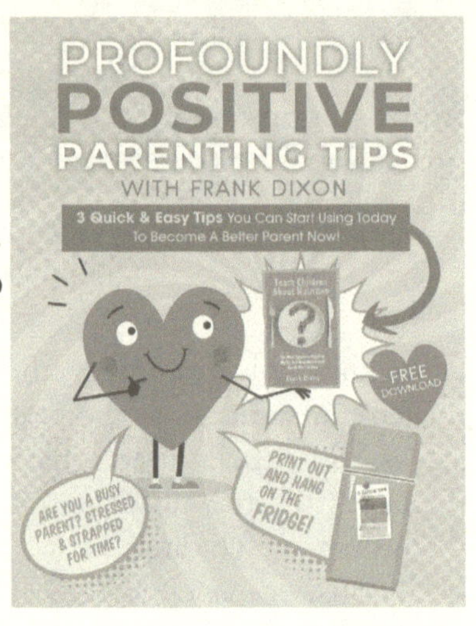

It's my gift to you, free of cost. Think of it as my way of saying thank you to you for purchasing this book.

Claim your download of Profoundly Positive Parenting with Frank Dixon by scanning the QR code below and join my mailing list.

Sign up below to grab your free copy, print it out and hang it on the fridge!

Sign Up By Scanning The QR Code With Your Phone's Camera To Be Redirected To A Page To Enter Your Email And Receive INSTANT Access To Your Download

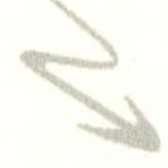
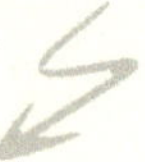

Before we jump in, I'd like to express my gratitude. I know this mustn't be the first book you came across and yet you still decided to give it a read. There are numerous courses and guides you could have picked instead that promise to make you an ideal and well-rounded parent while raising your children to be the best they can be.

But for some reason, mine stood out from the rest and this makes me the happiest person on the planet right now. If you stick with it, I promise this will be a worthwhile read.

In the pages that follow, you're going to learn the best parenting skills so that your child can grow to become the best version of themselves and in doing so experience a meaningful understanding of what it means to be an effective parent.

Notable Quotes About Parenting

"Children Must Be Taught How To Think, Not What To Think."

– Margaret Mead

"It's easier to build strong children than to fix broken men [or women]."

- Frederick Douglass

"Truly great friends are hard to find, difficult to leave, and impossible to forget."

– George Randolf

"Nothing in life is to be feared, it is only to be understood. Now is the time to understand more, so that we may fear less."

– Scientist Marie Curie

Table of Contents

Introduction

Although eating healthy is crucial in all phases of one's life, it is generally in early childhood when the brain, body, and strength are in their developmental phase. Children need a healthy and nutrient-rich diet—not just to ensure that they get all the vitamins, minerals, and nutrients required for healthy growth but also healthy mental and emotional growth. A balanced diet means stronger bones, a sharp mind, improved energy levels, and quality sleep, all of which affect our mood, productivity, and mental health.

A balanced ideal diet should include a wide array of nutritious foods belonging to different food groups. These include fruits and vegetables; whole grains; fat-free or low-fat dairy products; lean meats; beans and lentils; nuts and seeds, etc. According to the 2015–2020 Dietary Guidelines for Americans, individuals that take healthy foods in their diet are less prone to developing health conditions like heart disease, high blood pressure, diabetes, dental caries, osteoporosis, and cancer (U.S. Department of Health and Human Services; U.S. Department of Agriculture, 2015).

If we closely look at how a healthy diet impacts a child's life, we have many research studies that endorse the benefits. For example, a healthy diet is linked with improved cognitive functioning, especially memory and recall (Taras, 2005). Children that consume a nutrient-rich diet every day experience fewer mood swings (Hoyland et al., 2009). They are also less likely to skip school due to stomach and digestive problems (Rampersaud et al., 2005).

Our general eating habits are formed in the first few years of our lives. The right exposure and eating experiences shape our cravings for different textures, smells, and tastes. Poor nutrition increases the risk of developing health conditions like obesity in children which happens to be an already worrying dilemma. Encouraging young eaters to take charge of their health from an early age is a smart and beneficial strategy. When children are made aware of what good and bad foods are, they are more likely to stay away from junk food. When they are offered a variety of healthy treats and meals to choose from, they can keep their health in check and develop the habit of healthy eating. Speaking to them about how our meals affect our ability to learn and grow can serve as a promising lesson.

In this book, we are going to help both parents and young ones to take charge of their health by eating healthy; dismiss any nutrition myths they have about eating and certain foods; and learn how to raise healthy adults with a strong mind, better stamina, good energy levels, and improved well-being.

In the first few chapters, we go through the common struggles many parents face when trying to develop healthy eating habits. This is followed by a look into some prevailing eating disorders and myths around food. Then, we will dive further into what foods encourage healthy growth. Together, we can raise healthy adults who are ready to take charge of the world and prevent them from falling into the traps of unhealthy advertising and make sensible decisions about what to eat and what to abstain from.

Chapter 1:

You Don't Know My Child

Getting children to eat the things you want them to eat is no less than a nightmare for many parents. There are power struggles and temper tantrums because the greens don't taste good to them. The leafier the food, the more aversion toward it. When parents sense that the child isn't giving in, they do instead. They cave in by thinking at least something is going inside the child to fuel them for the day. But it wasn't always like this. If we go back a few decades, we remember our eating patterns and lifestyle. We didn't make faces, leave the table, or throw away our food. We sat and ate it like mature people, mostly because we feared staying hungry all night if we didn't eat it.

A modern parent doesn't believe in resorting to such harshness. They think of themselves as their child's friends. They are more compassionate and generous. This, in a way, takes away control from the parents because the child starts to believe that they have all the power in the relationship and, therefore, get away with their demands for takeout and junk foods. Where do children come up with the idea of what they want and when they want it?

Enter TV and online ads that are bombarded toward children offering deals after deals and discounts over a like, share, or comment. They see ads that promise them instant gratification and fancy toys on TV or their parent's phone, and they want it all. They see their favorite cartoons snacking on fries, burgers, and pizzas. When they go shopping with their parents, unhealthy food is marketed everywhere in the aisles to the final POS junctions in case they want to pick it up. Everywhere they go, unhealthy food choices surround them, be it the school, a friend's house, or a day at the park.

How can they want something other than that when they see it everywhere and find it readily available just a call/click away?

Moreover, there are many other reasons why parents allow their children to consume unhealthy meals and pack them lunches that are devoid of any healthy nutrients.

Why Parents Let Their Children Indulge in Unhealthy Foods

The biggest and most common reason, perhaps, is life getting in the way. Today, both parents have to work to pay the bills. From getting kids into good schools to ensuring a fluent lifestyle, they struggle to make ends meet. This wasn't the case before. In earlier times, men were considered the breadwinner of the house whereas the women were assigned the duty to look after the house and the kids. Also, organic food was readily available, and everything was cooked from scratch at home. Fresh vegetables, fruits, and spices were picked up from farms and sold in markets. The produce obtained was fresh and free of chemicals and pesticides. This isn't the case today.

With both parents working a full-time job, coming home with takeout meals and microwaving frozen foods seems much easier and doable. Cooking a healthy meal takes prep and cooking. With tiredness setting in and other obligations like putting kids to bed, folding the laundry, and cleaning the house are on the mind, free time becomes valuable. There is less mess in the kitchen, and therefore, parents don't have to worry about cleaning afterward.

But this shouldn't mean that your health has to suffer.

Then, there are picky eaters to worry about. As parents, we have all been there when our children barely touched their foods before claiming them as "yuck." We have seen lunch boxes come home unopened. We have had battles at mealtimes when children refuse to try something new you cooked. Other than the fact that your child may have some sensory issues, picky eating isn't a disorder: It's just a lack of convincing on the parent's part that leads to unadventurous eaters. When food is presented creatively, vegetables disguised and mashed with their favorite foods, picky eaters can still eat and remain healthy. When children don't get the opportunity to try something new and fresh, the parents think they are picky. In truth, they just become so used to the flavors and textures of certain foods that they naturally crave them all the time.

Another reason why children don't enjoy healthy alternatives is that they don't have a lot of them. According to a 2017 report by the Centers for Disease Control and Prevention (CDC), 90% of adults don't consume enough fruits and vegetables daily. How can you expect your child to pick up healthy eating if you don't feed them healthy foods? When parents insist on takeout and home deliveries, children normalize that behavior and develop the same eating patterns.

Yet unhealthy food is available everywhere and is comparatively cheaper than healthy alternatives. Take a gas station, for example. It sells everything from chips and drinks to chewing gum and ice cream. It isn't designed to, but it does. You won't ever find them stocking a salad or fruit in the store. Similarly, a salad costs more than a McDonald's Happy Meal these days. Add a few dollars, and you can upgrade the whole meal with larger fries and drink. As per recent numbers, there are approximately 13,673 McDonald's franchises in the United States alone (Statista, 2020). An average meal costs anywhere from $3 to $7, whereas a classic base salad begins from $8 to $15. With multiple kids to feed, a Happy Meal feels more doable and fulfilling than a salad with some leaves and vinaigrette.

Although they say that parenting isn't for the faint of heart, there is always so much that you can teach and learn from your kids. They weren't born with a craving for fries and burgers. They developed it because they had more of it. Had they been given a variety of fruits and vegetables to eat from, they would have appreciated the tastes and textures more. However, it isn't too late to turn the tables around and end the quest for pizzas, pasta, and chips. You can guide them about healthy eating options and instill good eating habits.

From Pizza, Pasta, and Chips to Fruits, Vegetables, and Proteins

Children don't naturally have an aversion toward healthy snacks. As stated earlier, it is the conditioning that happens with time. Whatever they are exposed to becomes their palate's favorite. Since reprogramming is possible and a necessity in times like today, here's how you can help them switch from wanting all the unhealthy treats to healthy ones.

Introduce wholesome and nutritious choices early on. When young, everything is experimentation for your child. They are curious and eager to know about the world they are in, and the same goes for what they eat. Developing a strong relationship with healthy foods, in the beginning, can form the habit of a lifetime.

Therefore, indulge their senses in a wide range of textures, smells, and tastes, so they have a variety to choose from. It may seem time-consuming, but if you take things strategically (i.e., plan) and prepare meals for the week beforehand, you can cut down on the amount of time needed to cook and serve. The more options they have on the dinner table, the more likely they will crave healthy foods. Good eating habits will allow them to enjoy different flavors and textures and grow healthy, too. Not to mention, the time that will be saved convincing your little one to take a bite of their vegetables.

Train the taste buds. Train them to enjoy different foods and be grateful for what they have. Show them how important eating healthy is and how thankful they should be to have their stomach full every day. When children start to view food as valuable, they will begin to respect it. They will also respect the needs of their body to stay healthy and fit.

Find healthier food alternatives. Who says you have to give them fried chips when you can bake or grill the same potatoes? Who says you have to give them ice cream when you can make a sorbet or fresh fruit smoothie at home? Why give them fried chicken instead of baked or grilled chicken? It tastes equally good. The point is, there are healthy substitutes for nearly every food. You can get bagels instead of pasties, or bake cakes at home with sugar substitutes. Since eliminating junk food is difficult, as kids are fond of it, try to cut back on it gradually and limit it to special days or events alone. On the other days, ensure that they enjoy the healthiest snacks and make healthy food choices as much as possible.

You can also give classic recipes a new makeover by substituting some ingredients with more tempting but healthy ones. Instead, you can add half white and brown sugar as opposed to all-white sugar in cakes, pastries, and desserts. Similarly, recipes that call for white bread can do the same with whole grain bread. Instead of deep-frying, you can resort to shallow or air-frying your chicken and savories. Instead of canned soups, broths, and dips, you can create your own with fresh ingredients without any chemicals or preservatives. The goal is to give recipes your touch of uniqueness and make them healthy.

Limit the consumption of sugary drinks and sodas. Avoid smoothies that contain ice cream and opt for ones that have yogurt in them. Try blending in bananas for sweetness with other fruits and vegetables so that they taste better, are thicker, and fulfilling. Put more emphasis on having fresh-squeezed juice blends of apples, beets, and carrots, as they are excellent immunity boosters. You can also add a splash of fresh lemon and cucumber to the water to give it some extra flavor.

As for ice cream, indulge in more frozen Popsicles made at home. Frozen treats are a child's favorite after-meal and afternoon snack. Why not make it healthy and nutritious? You can freeze fresh fruit juices, or add chunks of seasonal fruits to yogurts and freeze them into Popsicle trays.

Avoid getting store-bought, processed foods into your house. It may cut back on valuable time, but they give your child zero nutrients. With recipes of nearly every processed food online, you can make your nuggets, popcorn chicken, and Hot Pockets with cheese at home. The less packaged food in your house, the better. Doing so will help you focus on your child's overall diet rather than just specific foods.

Stop using food as a reward or bribe. We are all guilty of it. If you finish your vegetables, you can have ice cream after dinner. If you bring home the lunchbox empty, you can watch TV in the evening. If you finish your dinner, you can play with Daddy for a while before going to bed. Unintentionally, we have been ruining our children's appetite and eating habits with bribes and rewards. We promise them junk food in exchange for something we want them to do. This may seem like a good temporary solution but with a little pay-off in the longer run. Therefore, be mindful of what you promise in exchange for something and avoid bribing young kids with dreams of consuming unhealthy and sugary treats.

Disguise healthy foods with other foods. For example, when making a stew or broth, add a helping of greens to bring more flavors. Mash vegetables like carrots and peas with mashed potatoes. Add some freshly cut fruits like apples and pineapples to salads to add some sweetness. If children don't enjoy eating fruits on their own, juice them with other juices or add a sweet dip with them to make them more tempting.

Restaurants don't use the freshest ingredients in their dishes. They usually go for cheaper, more readily available products. Some aren't even cleaned properly. Then there is also the case of reusing leftover cooking oil, poultry, and meat. Reheating the oil and frying things in it can be hazardous for your child's health. Restaurant takeout meals are also full of unhealthy fats and added sugars which is why it is ideal that you cook at home. You can stock up on some fresh fruits and vegetables, and after cutting them, freeze them until further use. You can do the same for soups, poultry, and meat. Doing so will cut down on the time needed to make a meal from scratch. If you are a working parent, you can plan your meals and do most of the cutting and chopping over the weekends. You can also make food in large batches so that it can be reused later.

When going grocery shopping, get the kids involved. Make a list of items that you need from the store and hand them to your child. Make sure to add more fresh produce like seasonal fruits, vegetables, and meat. Teach the child how to shop for the freshest fruits and vegetables by smelling and feeling their textures. You can also guide them on how to read labels so that they become aware of what they are putting in themselves. Basic knowledge about calories and added sugars in their favorite foods and drinks will make them ponder over their food choices, as the consequences include obesity, gas, bloating, and unwanted weight gain.

Finally, if you want your child to eat healthier and nutrient-rich foods, make them visibly available in your house. Usually, when children get hungry, they rush to the kitchen and walk toward the fridge. Make sure they find lots of healthy options to pick from. Similarly, if you want them to intentionally eat healthy, you can also keep fruits in their sight to trigger a craving. As for less nutritious items, store them away in a cabinet or drawer they rarely open. It is best to avoid bringing such foods into your house, as they will trigger a craving. Make it a habit to eat less nutritious snacks only when outside.

Chapter 2:

Healthy Eating: What It Is and Why It's Important

Eating healthy benefits individuals in all steps of life. When we are young and growing, healthy eating enriches our system with the much-needed nutrients necessary for proper development. As we grow older and start school, our level of activity and engagement increases, so there is a need for more vitamins, minerals, and healthy foods. When we enter professional stages, healthy foods help us remain focused, attentive, and productive. They fuel our system with the right energy needed to get through the day. This goes on and on. Although eating healthily is a decision one can take in any phase of their life, starting a healthy lifestyle early on can have long-term benefits. Healthy eating in the formative years of childhood makes a child more likely to stick with healthy eating as they become adults.

In this regard, a promising health initiative called MyPlate was introduced by the former First Lady Michelle Obama. The guide helped parents monitor their child's food intake and encourage the creation of healthy eating habits.

Healthful eating involves the consumption of a variety of nutritious foods. The idea is to incorporate foods from various food groups into your child's meal so that they can have a well-rounded diet. In the MyPlate initiative, parents are advised to divide the child's plate into four sections. It should include fruits, vegetables, grains, and proteins. On the side of the plate should be a glass representing dairy. MyPlate advises parents that a child's diet should limit foods with excess fats and sugars; these should be occasional foods and only consumed once in a while.

This is what healthful eating is all about!

You replace foods high in trans fats, sugar, and added salts with healthy, organically produced, and fresh ingredients. Following such a diet has a ton of benefits from improved focus to stronger bones. In this chapter, we will look at these in detail and learn about the nine food groups essential for a child in their growing years.

What Does a Healthy Diet Do for Your Child?

Most parents think that letting children eat whatever they want, whenever they want, is the best way to encourage eating. There are little to no rules around the dinner table. Children are allowed to reject what's on their plate and demand something unhealthy. Or worse, they are bribed with promises about unhealthy junk foods so that they can finish their vegetables. However, this isn't how healthy eating habits take form. There have to be some rules, stringent ones, to ensure healthy eating habits from the get-go. Surely, this next section will have you convinced why your child needs to eat healthily and why now is the best time to start setting healthy expectations around food.

Healthy eating improves the functioning of the heart. With heart diseases as the leading cause of death throughout the world, it shouldn't come as a surprise that food and unhealthy habits around food are the biggest culprits to blame. Nearly half of U.S. adults have some form of cardiovascular disease, as per the American Heart Association (Benjamin et al., 2019), with high blood pressure or hypertension as the most worrying concern. Hypertension or high blood pressure can result in a stroke, heart attack, or heart failure. Did you know that some resources cite that it is possible to prevent 8% of premature strokes and heart diseases with lifestyle changes that include healthy eating and increased physical activity (Shan et al., 2020)? The right foods can keep cholesterol levels, blood pressure, and blood sugar levels in control, ensuring that the heart stays healthy.

Then, there is also increased immunity to think about. Stronger immunity means fewer trips to the hospital due to flu, colds, and fevers. Seasonal fruits and vegetables packed with vitamins A, B, C, and D promote stronger immunity. According to one study focusing on the health of children in 11 Latin American countries, a high intake of fruits and vegetables reduced the risk of rhinoconjunctivitis in children that causes red eyes, nasal congestion, and skin conditions like eczema (Cepeda et al., 2017).

Healthful eating is also linked with improved mood. In a 2016 study, researchers concluded that diets high in glycemic load cause triggering of symptoms of fatigue and depression (Breymeyer et al., 2016). A diet high in glycemic load includes one that has refined carbs. These are most commonly found in our favorite soft drinks, cakes, cookies, bread, etc. On the other hand, fruits, vegetables, and whole grains have a low glycemic load. These foods are known to improve mood and health.

A healthy diet also means improved memory for your child. As they start school, they are going to need all their brain power to learn and absorb new concepts and information. A healthy diet helps with cognition and memory. Preparing for exams and doing well in them becomes a possibility for children when their body's needs are taken care of. According to a 2015 study, certain foods high in vitamin C, D, and E improve memory (Dominguez & Barbagallo, 2018). Foods like fish, which are high in omega-3 fatty acids, are also an example. Such foods improve recall and help with the processing of information. They also load the body with optimal energy, ensuring that the mind remains focused and attentive throughout the day. Moreover, children that don't receive an adequate amount of iron and iodine in their diets experience cognitive delays, cognitive decline, and delays in motor development.

Lastly, children that consume a sufficient amount of calcium and magnesium in their diets have stronger bones and teeth. Strong bones reduce the chances of bone-related injuries and issues like osteoporosis and arthritis in adults.

7 Must-Eat Nutrients for Your Child

Whether you have a picky eater, a try-anything type young one, or a snacker that sticks with junk food, the right nutrients will help them grow into healthy and fit adults. It is a no-brainer that children go through the most important developmental changes from the ages of before they hit teenage years. Their brain develops at a fast rate, their body changes in different ways, and their mental cognition and understanding about how things work starts to happen. No wonder they are always hungry! Luckily, healthy eating can fuel those changes. What constitutes healthy eating and what nutrients or food groups are composed of will be explained below.

Protein

Proteins help with the breakdown of food into energy. Proteins build muscles, help the body fight infection, and make it easier for the body to transport oxygen.

Broths, stews, and lean cuts of meat are digestible by the body and therefore encouraged to give to young kids. Food high in protein includes meat, fish, poultry, eggs, beans, dairy, and nuts. Ideally, a growing child needs about three to five ounces of protein per day. For older children, the amount goes up to five to eight ounces.

Fats

Healthy fats are an excellent source of energy for young children. Fats prevent hunger pangs and keep the body fueled with energy throughout the day by storing it. Fats are essential to help the body use the nutrients properly. Foods that are rich in healthy fats include whole milk products, fish, meat, cooking oils, and nuts. Medical experts suggest that a growing child's diet should primarily consist of 30% of unsaturated fats (Bernstein, 2016).

Calcium

The calcium found mostly in dairy products like milk, yogurt, cheeses, and tofu helps with making the bones stronger and healthier. Parents that ensure regular intake of milk in their child's diet can rest assured that their child will have strong teeth and a sturdy structure. Bone-related injuries and conditions are becoming common among adults these days. This can be prevented if young children are given as little as one cup of milk every day. Calcium helps with blood clotting, heart function, and proper muscle flexibility.

Generally, children aged four to eight should receive 1000 milligrams of calcium per day (Bernstein, 2016).

Iron

Like calcium, iron is also an important food group. It helps the body circulate blood carrying oxygen in the cells. Foods that contain high levels of iron include red meat, poultry, liver, whole grains, beans, shellfish, and iron-fortified cereals. Children should receive 10 milligrams of iron per day (Bernstein, 2016).

Fiber

Fiber promotes healthy bowel regularity in children. Constipation, diarrhea, stomachaches, and other gut-related issues are common among school-age children. Lack of proper sleep, unhealthy eating, and a sedentary lifestyle can all cause bowel problems. The fiber in a child's diet can prevent that. Furthermore, it also reduces the chances of heart diseases and cancers. Foods that are rich in fiber include chickpeas, whole-grain cereals, kidney beans, seeds, lentils, and some nuts.

Vitamin C

Like vitamin D, vitamin C is another important vitamin. Fruits and vegetables enriched with vitamin C help fight seasonal flu and colds. They keep the body's cells together, help with quick recovery of wounds, build stronger bones, and strengthen the walls of blood vessels. Foods that contain vitamin C include all citrus fruits like oranges, lemons, and limes, as well as strawberries, cabbage, potatoes, melons, tomatoes, spinach, mango, cauliflower, etc. A child aged four to eight needs 25 milligrams of vitamin C per day. A child older than that needs 45 milligrams of vitamin C per day (Bernstein, 2016).

Vitamin D

Vitamin D is vital for the development of healthy bones and teeth. It also promotes good hair and skin health. Although it is rarely found in foods, it can be added to several dairy products and cereals. Sunlight is the most obvious and promising source of vitamin D which is why you should encourage your young ones to get outside and play during the hours when the sun is out. However, be sure to not allow too much direct exposure, as there is some evidence of it causing skin cancer. Ideally speaking, a growing child needs 600 international units (IU) of vitamin D per day (Bernstein, 2016).

Chapter 3:

Eating Disorders and Unhealthy Eating Patterns

As children grow older and come face-to-face with the many challenges life throws at them, their preferences around food also change. There comes a time when they become cautious about their weight, height, and skin. To avoid getting fat or developing acne and other skin-related conditions, they omit certain food groups altogether or consume more than one or two. Both of these conditions are unhealthy and can lead to the development of unhealthy eating habits and disorders.

Since young children are smaller in stature and weight, even a slight change in their weight due to refusal of certain foods can trigger an eating disorder. By the time parents become aware of it, the child has developed an eating disorder and has trouble switching to a more balanced eating style.

Eating disorders in preteens and teenagers could cause serious physical problems if left untreated. Unlike weight loss, one can't overcome an eating disorder with sheer willpower alone. Most of the time, a child needs proper medical treatment and therapy to restore healthy eating habits and weight.

A Look at the Most Common Eating Disorders Among Children

There is little information as to what triggers an eating disorder. As per many various research studies, they are a combination of behavioral, biological, and social factors. The biggest factor is a thirst for recognition and validation among teenagers. With social media apps like Facebook, Instagram, and Snapchat rewarding youngsters with instant gratification in the form of likes and pleasant comments, there is a constant battle of who looks the best and why.

Body image issues are becoming more common and worrying. Young girls who are thin resort to unhealthy eating behaviors so that they can look more pleasant. Young men, with their hormones raging, want to look cool and indulge in rigorous exercise regimens to build muscles and stamina. To cope with the increasing pressure and competition to look a certain way, children and youngsters engage in harmful eating habits that go hand in hand with many psychiatric problems like depression, anxiety, and substance abuse.

Below are four of the most prevalent eating disorders among teenagers and children in their prime growing years.

Anorexia Nervosa

Anorexia nervosa is a condition in which children, especially teenagers, try to maintain a weight that is below average for their height and age. They do so out of intense fear of gaining weight or becoming fat. This happens when they have a distorted vision of what an ideal body image is and perceive themselves as fat—even when they are lean and skinny.

To ensure that they remain underweight, children with anorexia intentionally starve themselves. They sparsely eat and purge food by using laxatives or self-induced vomiting. They lack guidance and recognize how their actions lead to unwanted medical emergencies. As a parent, you can begin to notice the signs when they stop eating or have little of everything. You can also note how they constantly speak about getting fat or being anxious about not fitting into their clothes. They may also request to join a difficult and hardcore workout regimen and put their body and bones under a lot of unwanted stress. Thinning of hair, discoloration of fingers due to lack of oxygen, soft hair covering the body, dizziness, fatigue, insomnia, fainting, and absence of menstruation in girls are all signs to watch out for.

Bulimia Nervosa

Bulimia nervosa is an eating disorder in which a child engages in episodes of binging and purging, meaning there are days when they won't stop eating followed by days where they will try to get rid of every extra calorie in their body by restricting themselves. Examples of purging include voluntary vomiting or excessive exercise. Bulimia is more common among women in their teens. The patients suffer from other mental health issues as well such as stress, anxiety, substance abuse, or depression. When left untreated, patients can engage in self-harming behaviors.

The most visible symptoms include calluses on knuckles and the back of the hands; stained or discolored teeth; cases of self-induced vomiting; weight fluctuations; swelling in the jaw area and cheeks; and irregular menstrual cycles.

Avoidant/Restrictive Food Intake Disorder (ARFID)

In this type of eating disorder, a child refuses to or is unable to eat certain foods based on their taste, aroma, texture, or temperature. Many children despise the taste of broccoli, and no matter how much their parents try to feed them or disguise them with other vegetables, their stomachs just can't digest it. This eating disorder can lead to inadequate growth in children, nutritional deficiencies, weight loss, and impaired psychosocial functioning. This can be damaging to your child's health in the long run, especially if they restrict eating an important nutrient or food group. Also, the child may refuse to eat foods of the same color and texture, assuming they will taste the same.

Binge Eating Disorder

Children and teenagers who develop the disorder of binge eating consume large amounts of food often and in secret. Eating provides them a means of escape from sadness, boredom, or depression. They will eat when someone in their class doesn't reciprocate the feelings they have for them. They will eat when they fail an exam and worry that they will get expelled. They eat when they want to lose weight but can't do so despite trying, and all the emotions and feelings of helplessness overtake them. Children seldom tell anyone about what they are doing because they feel embarrassed or guilty about it. However, the compulsion is so strong that they can't stop.

Just because someone binge eats doesn't mean they will be overweight or obese. Even children with average weight do it. Binge eating is often the result of some trauma, hurtful encounter, or depression. Stress can also induce binge eating symptoms in children.

Chapter 4:

Breaking Bad Eating Habits

The triggering of an eating disorder doesn't take place on its own. There are both mental and medical reasons behind it. Since they don't come off with a ton of noticeable symptoms, it is hard for both parents and children to spot them and recover on their own. Treatment is required along with consistent support from the family. As for a parent, your job is to closely monitor your child's daily food intake and their attitude around food. Have their eating patterns changed? Are they restoring to old, unhealthy eating practices? Are they changing their behavior around food or not? Are they eating healthy foods from all food groups?

These are all questions that can help you understand where your child stands in terms of the disorder and how easy or difficult it is to snap them out of it. This calls for some clever strategies along with tracking their food consumption. Know that breaking out of bad habits isn't difficult, given the child is guided throughout. There has to be a balance between empathy and authoritativeness. You may find it tempting to back off to avoid any power struggles, but it is your child in question. Whether they agree or not, you are their sole guardian until they are legally old enough to take care of themselves. When making new rules or setting structures, remember that your child didn't choose to develop an eating disorder. They developed it out of some pressure or stress. Your goal is to address that first and then help your child overcome the disorder.

Getting Started: The Right Mindset Matters

Below are some tips and ideas to ensure that your child eats healthy and overcomes their eating disorder.

Avoid dieting in front of your child or request them to start one. Unless their pediatrician suggests something like a routine diet to get in shape, there is no need to push them to start one. Allow them the chance to eat when they are hungry and stop when they feel full. Don't make them finish everything on their plate when they repeatedly tell you that they can't have more. Children are young and naive. They don't sugarcoat things as we do. If they say they are full, they probably are. Even if they are lying, they will soon ask for something when they feel the urge to eat. Also, avoid going on fad diets in front of your child, as it sends them the message that you don't love the way you are.

There are, of course, healthier ways of getting fit and maintaining a healthy weight.

Have conversations with your child about healthy and unhealthy food choices. If they are old enough to understand what calories are and what foods have more of them, they should be able to understand why they should restrict their diet to the amount that they can easily burn off.

You can also encourage them to form a healthy relationship with their food. This is possible if they stop viewing some foods as good and others bad. This sets up cravings as well as guilt after they consume something that their parents labeled as bad food. When you try to break an unhealthy eating habit, forbidding some foods is only going to cause more problems. The restricted foods will automatically become more tempting. The best way to go about it instead is to have more of the foods that you want your child to consume in the house. When your child doesn't find a less nutritious snack in the house, they are going to crave it less.

Emphasize talking about how to eat. This is often an ignored topic in households. We are socially inclined to finish off our plates. From infancy, we have been forced to clean our plates. This practice needs to change, and children should have the power to decide when they feel full. There should also be no shaming when the child requests another helping.

Children tend to eat more during the day. There is more actively involved, and therefore, there is a faster digestion rate. Don't limit their food intake by setting stringent eating hours. Also, be patient when the child starts to like or dislike some particular food. Don't force-feed; try to disguise the food with other foods.

Cultivate a positive body image, and talk about how your child shouldn't feel forced to lose or gain weight because of what others tell them. If they feel happy about how they look, that is all that should matter. There are many other ways to make your child feel good about their body. For example, you can teach about acceptance. Everyone has a different body type and shape, and we are all beautifully different. Your child should accept that they own their individuality. You can talk to them about the many wonderful things their body does for them and how food is the right way to reward it. Talk to them about the functioning and responsibility of various organs and how they can help support their optimal functioning by eating healthy. You can also encourage physical activity and movement. The more they move around, the less time their body will have to store excess fat. However, make sure that they find those activities and work out fun to do.

Don't ever tease, criticize, or pass a comment about their appearance. Many parents feel that by shaming their kids, they are doing them a big favor. This isn't how you motivate someone to change a bad habit or preference. You need to be supportive on their journey to healthy weight maintenance and help them reach their desired weight goal. Judging and criticizing won't do much: They already get that from everyone else.

Encourage self-esteem and self-worth to cope with school-related pressures and expectations. If there is one thing that movies and TV shows have taught us, it is this: A fat child or teenager will never be the central character. They will always get side roles and rarely get a solid script or any quality screen time. No one wants to be friends with them or eat lunch with them. They are constantly bullied by a bunch of mean children and never have a fairy-tale happy ending. Their life only starts to matter when they lose weight, learn how to dress and do their makeup… PERIOD.

It's unfair and sets the wrong expectations. When your child sees a movie depicting a similar story line, they feel like they are expected to do the same. They must lose weight to be recognized and seen. Losing weight will ensure that they aren't bullied, have friends, and hopefully have someone to go to prom with. Encourage them to be assertive and say no if they feel that they are mistreated by their friends. Show them how they can better express their needs and wants and decide what's best for them. Have conversations about the messages TV shows and movies depict and how they need to be revised and changed.

Chapter 5:

Are You Serious?

The reason we find parenting challenges in the first place is because there is a lot of guilt involved when something goes wrong: "I should have given them the sweater to take on with them to school; they would have never gotten that cold." "I should have read the labels more carefully before buying that product." "I must learn how to cook better so that my child starts to eat properly."

Parents feel especially challenged when it comes to knowing what to feed their children. Despite the vast range of information available, it always comes down to personal experiences from those who have successfully raised healthy and happy children. We find our parents as the best guide when it comes to any problem related to parenting. We turn to them for advice and guidance.

However, not all advice you receive is relevant or good. Some can be misleading and untrue. What might have worked for your parents with you may not work for you and your child. It's a different kind of bond and need. Today's children are more independent and vocal about their preferences. Many external forces shape their decisions and food choices. Advertising also has a major role to play. Today's kids are more exposed to ads and creative marketing campaigns that urge them to be a part of them. There is also social pressure to worry about. When all your child's friends bring store-bought lunches to school, sooner or later, your child will demand the same.

First up, you aren't the only struggling parent here. How to get children to eat healthy and develop good eating habits is every parent's predicament. On one hand, it is difficult to sift through all the advice that you receive from friends, family, and the Internet. Understandably, you want the best for your child, but what can you do when they won't give in to eating fruits and vegetables?

Having fussy eaters at home makes for another challenging feat. Some children have distinct tastes and like to assert their dominance and identity with what they eat. The first step is to decipher fact from fiction. You need to debunk any and all myths regarding nutrition. It is time to give up on make-believe concepts and clear misconceptions around your child's diet and food.

Common Myths About Child Nutrition and How to Debunk Them

Speaking of myths, the biggest and possibly the most common myth around child nutrition is that parents believe if their child skips a meal, they will starve to death. This isn't the case. Children are intuitive eaters. They know what they want when they want it. Even before their birth, they have been following a structure. Their demand for food has only increased since then. As they grow older and become more vocally capable, they show excellent expression toward it.

As a parent, don't feel guilty about your child skipping a meal. They aren't just as hungry as you thought. They may still have some energy left from the last meal that doesn't trigger hunger. Wait for them to come to you and ask to be fed. If they are older and fully able to feed themselves, simply ensure that they can find something nutritious to munch on when they have an urge. That is how you can incorporate healthy foods into their diet.

Other than this, here are some myths around child nutrition and how you can debunk them.

Myth: All kids dislike vegetables.

Again, it isn't true. Many children enjoy eating vegetables. It is more about the kind of exposure they have. As parents, try to experiment with various foods, especially vegetables from early on. When children are naive, they rely on what textures feel good and what foods taste good. Their primary concern isn't whether it's a vegetable or not. The more choices they are offered, the more diverse their palate will be.

Luckily, there are tons of ways to cook vegetables. They can be sautéed in some olive oil, air-fried, deep-fried with batter, and presented as side dishes with meats and poultry. There are uncountable salads you can make with them. You can also juice some produce like carrots, beets, lemons, etc. You can also add leafy vegetables in fruit blends to give them a bit of a unique taste and color.

Myth: Don't bother serving food again that your child rejected.

The taste of something isn't the only reason a child rejects something. It could have been an abnormal blend of spices, rawness of textures, or a lack of hunger that causes your child to reject eating something. You must continue to experiment and incorporate the same food in other dishes but cooked differently to know for sure. You never know: They may like it all the more when it's cooked differently. For example, a child will be more than happy to eat fries but won't show the same enthusiasm when presented with mashed potatoes. Similarly, chicken cooked in curry may not tempt your child, but fried chicken might. This means that there is always a possibility that the food alone isn't to blame for the rejection. Keep on trying and experimenting by giving recipes a makeover so that your child continues to eat healthy—one way or another.

Myth: A multivitamin a day gives my child all the nutrients they need.

This is another common myth about child nutrition. No matter how many multivitamins your child takes, the truth remains the same: Consumption from natural sources and foods is still the best. This misconception prevents parents from giving their children adequate nutrition for healthy growth. Let's remember from this day forward that multivitamins are not a food substitute. They simply enhance natural food intake. Your child still benefits from natural resources like fortified products, plants, and animals.

Therefore, focus more on getting them to eat the fresh, locally sourced, and organic products as much as possible. If you have a garden space, you can even grow your own vegetables and fruits.

Myth: Sugar gets children into hyperactive mode.

Sugars offer children zero nutritional value. Sugar addiction is a real problem, and the sooner parents realize this, the better. This addiction is known to lead to several behavioral issues like mood swings. If they naturally have a sweet tooth, there are many substitutes like fruits and nuts. Sugar doesn't necessarily make your child hyperactive. They cause an immediate blood sugar drop since they are digested quickly. This can leave the child feeling irritated and distracted. What they need is a healthy and balanced diet with foods that contain natural and healthy sugars so that they can remain active throughout the day.

Myth: All kids should eat three meals a day.

It is similar to the first myth around child nutrition that we talked about. To further stress how wrong it is, you must know that your child's stomach is the size of their fist. They can only fit a certain amount of food at a given time. Their bellies aren't designed to handle three big meals. Besides, there is also the curious case of how digestion works. Some foods take longer to break down and release energy whereas some are digested quickly. You can always rely on smaller, more frequent meals throughout the day to ensure that your child keeps eating healthily. But snacking should only be allowed when the snacks are healthy and nutritious; otherwise, it can lead to child obesity which is a pressing concern these days. Think carrots, cheese slices, fresh juices, and fruit salads as snacks.

Myth: Juice is a great way to give my child the desired nutrients.

It's true that some form of nutrients and minerals is better than none but thinking that juicing vegetables and fruits is an ideal way for it is wrong. Juicing isn't essential. When fruits and vegetables are chopped down and blended to form juices, the nutrients and fiber bonds also break. This breakage takes away the essence it had. Juicing reduces the fiber content in fruits and vegetables and also increases the sugar content in them.

Myth: My child won't get fat if I feed them nonfat foods.

Untrue: Your child will get fat if they are being constantly fed food of any kind. Excess of anything is bad. Even fruits, vegetables, meat, and dairy products have calories and sugar in them. In adequate quantities, they do all the good you expect them to, but when consumed in large quantities, they can cause weight fluctuations. Healthy fats extracted from nuts, seeds, lean meats, and olive oil nourish the developing brain of a child. It makes them feel satiated after a meal. Fats are usually rich in flavor and taste. If a child doesn't feel full after a meal, they may rely on additional, non-healthy snacks to fill their stomachs. This will lead to weight gain and poor metabolism.

Therefore, encourage the intake of healthy fats and guide children about what foods are healthy and unhealthy to consume.

Myth: I have no power over what my teenager eats. They are old enough to decide, aren't they?

No matter how old they grow, they will always remain your little one. The key is education about nutrition. It has to start at home. You may not have any control over their eating habits and choices, but you can help mold them from the start. If they are school-going children, you still have the chance to prepare two meals for them in a day. Make sure they are full of nutritional value and taste. As for lunch that they buy from outside, promote the idea of a well-balanced diet. Become a role model yourself. If they notice that you munch on some hot dog or chips at work, they are going to develop the same habits.

Myth: My child skips breakfast often, but that's okay because they eat a healthy lunch and dinner.

Breakfast is the first and most important meal of the day. Children need to perform at their best in the first few hours of the day when they are at school or play. They need to have the stamina to get through the day which can only be offered via a healthy breakfast. If carving out time for breakfast is difficult, you can always prepare some on-the-go healthy treats they can eat on their way to school. This can include overnight oats; egg and ham sandwiches; whole grain toast; or hard-boiled eggs. You can even cut up fruits that can easily be consumed in the car or on the school bus.

Myth: I should only give my child fresh fruits and veggies.

Anything fresh is indeed better than packed goods. However, in places where only some fruits and vegetables are available year-round, you can use frozen and packed versions of them. The reason is because frozen fruits and vegetables are packed when they are at their peak ripeness (i.e., most nutritious). You don't need to go to the store for that. You can purchase directly from a local farm during the peak season and buy the product in bulk. Then, you can slice them and freeze them for later use. This way, you can have fruits like strawberries and vegetables like okra year-round.

Myth: I must give my child extra carbs because they engage in a lot of sports.

If you give your child a well-balanced diet all year, you don't need to change when they are training for a big sports event. They don't need the extra carbs to load up on because of a big game. Carbs take time to digest and fuel the body with promised energy. Giving them right before a big game won't do any good, as the body won't start processing it until later.

What you can do instead is give them a good mix of protein and carbs throughout the day, so they can remain energized throughout the day. If they have a big game the next morning, you can add in some pasta or potatoes at dinner so that their body sustains that energy. This should be enough.

Myth: It's a parent's job to ensure that the child eats well.

Children indeed learn all the good and bad habits from their parents and siblings. They see and mimic their actions, behaviors, and attitudes. However, to solely blame the parent when the child doesn't want to eat healthy foods is wrong. There can be a hundred reasons why a child may avoid eating healthy foods. They may simply not like the taste of them or crave other things. It comes down to how they are guided and mentored. Having healthy conversations about how food affects our body, mind, and mood is a great topic to initiate the development of healthy eating habits. As soon as the child becomes aware of what they should and shouldn't eat, they will begin to take responsibility for what they intake. They will also become cautious about excess consumption of anything. The right role models and guidance can make them make sensible decisions about their food preferences and choices.

Myth: A few bites of healthy foods should be enough, right?

Did you know some studies suggest that a child's liking and disliking toward a certain food group determines how it will be absorbed in the body? This means that you need to stop force-feeding your child this instant, as it won't do them any good if they don't like it. You can always present a certain food in different ways. For example, if a child doesn't like eating apples, you can add thin slices of them in salads and desserts. You can also juice a few chunks with other juices and mask their taste. You can caramelize them and make a homemade marmalade with strawberries or oranges. That way, they will continue to eat normally and not even know about it.

Myth: I can always give my child more fruits to compensate for the lack of vegetables.

Every food has unique properties, nutrients, and vitamins. They are all absorbed by the body in different ways. Therefore, thinking that one food can serve as a substitute for another is wrong. Fruits are sweet, so they are easy to feed to children. However, they lack the phytochemicals that most vegetables contain. Phytochemicals fuel the body with energy and prevent cells from damage that could lead to cancers. Ideally, you should give your child food from all food groups and try not to omit any. Again, you can use the disguising strategy to mask the taste and scent of certain foods.

Chapter 6:

Healthy Eating for the Mind

Our bodies function in the same way a machine does. They need fuel and energy to run optimally. The right fuels hold the power to positively or negatively impact their performance. What your child eats and drinks doesn't only shape their body type but also affects their mood, focus, and productivity levels. Nutrition plays a key role in how attentive, vigilant, and energized we are throughout the day. Different foods have different abilities to provide the body with a surge of energy when it needs it the most. We know we need a coffee the minute we wake up because of the long day ahead. Add to that a bunch of kids to worry about, and no amount of coffee in the world can keep you as energized as you wish you could be.

Some foods like refined carbohydrates, abundant in simple sugars, promise a quick boost of energy. Other foods like meat, legumes, and starchy food need more time for digestion and energy release. The right foods also impact our well-being and emotions. Have you ever noticed how eating some ice cream from the tub makes everything a little better?

In this next chapter, we look at how food can help children build focus, stamina, and attention. The focus is on giving them foods that will boost their concentration levels and memory so that they do well in exams and stay healthy.

How Certain Foods Improve Focus, Productivity, and Attention

Maintaining focus and concentration is imperative for children in their developmental ages. School and academic challenges can be a lot for children who feel mentally fatigued or distracted. Not only do they have a difficult time understanding, but they also fail to do well in exams. Although there are many strategies like mindfulness and attention-building exercises, not many parents know that food is also a major contributor to building focus and attention. The brain uses 20% of the energy produced by the body in a day (Richardson, 2019). This means that you need to eat properly to give your brain a chance to perform at its optimal best. Children who don't receive the desired nutrients that build memory and attention could develop poor recall, delay in the interpretation of the received information, and concentration issues.

"But how does eating the right foods come into play?"

It all starts with what you eat. When the body digests food, it gets split into its basic components. Of these, proteins and fats are utilized by the body to rebuild tissue and dissolve micronutrients. Carbohydrates help the brain with providing energy.

When carbohydrates are broken down, they turn into glucose: its most basic form. The brain feeds on this glucose. Since different foods have different ways and rates at which they break down, it can take a while for the sugar to kick in and work its magic. Simple carbohydrates break down at a faster rate and rush glucose throughout the bloodstream. This leaves the child with a short-lived but strong boost of attention and energy. They become alert, more focused, and attentive. Complex carbohydrates—found most commonly in whole grains, fruits, and vegetables—take longer to break down and release glucose steadily in several hours which is ideal if the goal is to maintain a steady focus like that needed in exams.

Evidence suggests that a regular intake of fruits and vegetables in the diet isn't just good for the body but also for the mind. In one paper, researchers identify which foods affect our day-to-day experiences and mood. In the study, a group of participants reported their food consumption, behaviors, and mood over 13 days. Researchers evaluated how their food choices affected their daily experiences. The findings revealed that the more fruits and vegetables people consumed, the more engaged, creative, and happy they were than those who took a limited amount of these complex carbohydrates in their diet (Conner et al., 2015).

The researchers believed this could be because fruits and vegetables contain important nutrients that promote the production of dopamine in the body. Dopamine is a neurotransmitter that enables us to be curious, motivated, happy, and engaged. It also releases antioxidants that help improve memory, minimize inflammation, and cause a positive impact on our mood. This means that if you want your child to be their best, feel happiest, and be inquisitive and creative, make decisions around their food choice sensibly. When they learn to eat healthy, they won't have as many cravings as before.

Ideal Foods to Incorporate in Your Child's Diet

No one would put olive oil in their car to make it run. Similarly, your body doesn't need shakes, iced lattes, and chocolate milk to run efficiently. Food has an incredible power to affect your memory, mental clarity, and mood. Additionally, it helps build focus and improve productivity. If it affects your mood and focus, it can do the same for your child who needs it more. Unlike you, they rely solely on their focus and attention to grasp new information. They can't rationalize things on their own and take in what they receive. If they are young, they can't differentiate between right and wrong. They need your guidance, empathy, and support. When it comes to food choices, once again, they rely on your guidance and the example you set.

Ultimately, what foods can you offer them to boost their ability to focus, remain undistracted, and sharp? Here are 10 items to help answer this question:

Water

You may not categorize water as a food, but it is one of the most important drinks and also the most overlooked. Drinking adequate amounts of water enhances brain function. The brain is 85% water. Water provides the brain with the electrical energy it needs to function at its best. A child's brain needs twice the energy as other cells that make up the body. The production of dopamine and norepinephrine, responsible for improved executive functioning and hormone regulation, all depends on the amount of water they drink. In one study, drinking sufficient water allows you to think faster by 14%, be more creative, and remain focused for longer ("Eating your way to focus and concentration," 2017).

Beets

Beets are packed with healthy nitrates that promote the conversion into nitric oxide, a component that improves blood flow, lowers blood pressure, and dilates your blood vessels. Increased blood flow is a sign that your brain is receiving more oxygen and nutrient-rich blood. Children may not be tempted to eat raw beets on their own. You can juice them and add them to salads or smoothies for some excellent color and sweetness. Research shows that eating beets improves cognitive function in the frontal lobe of the brain (Clifford et al., 2015). This is the region where most of the focus-related activity happens.

Dark Chocolate

What kid doesn't love chocolate? Did you know that dark chocolate, not the sugary and milky kind, builds focus in many ways? First, it has a similar composition as that of caffeine which is an instant alertness booster. Second, it contains magnesium that helps one de-stress. Magnesium also releases endorphins and serotonin in the body that enlightens your mood (Santiago-Rodríguez et al., 2018).

Eggs

Proteins found in eggs are an excellent source of energy that keeps the stomach full for several hours. Research shows that eating eggs daily is linked with improved mental energy, better emotional processing, and faster reaction times—three things your child can take advantage of (Mohajeri et al., 2015). Unless your child has intolerance toward it or is on a completely vegetarian diet, incorporate eggs in their diet to provide them with healthy nutrients. There are tons of ways you can add an egg to their diet. From hard-boiled to sunny-side up eggs; in cakes and pudding batters; in omelets; and as a side dish to your mains, there are so many different ways you can increase your child's egg consumption.

Blueberries

Research has shown that adding blueberries to your diet can protect against brain damage caused by free radicals. It also reduces the chances of one developing brain-related health conditions like dementia and Alzheimer's disease. Blueberries are rich in antioxidants that improve muscle function as well as learning. Blueberries have a unique taste. They are great in blends and smoothies as well as toppings on desserts and ice cream. If you want to stick to health-conscious and simple recipes, give your child a bowl of blueberries in yogurt (Nolasco, 2014).

Bananas

Have you ever watched athletes munch on a banana during a break? It's because bananas are full of energy. They are easy, delicious, and naturally sweet. They can make you alert and attentive within a short time. According to a 2008 study, students who consumed a banana before an exam did better than those that didn't. Researchers monitored their performance and reviewed it with the performance of those who didn't eat a banana. It was evident that students that ate a banana had put more thought and devotion into solving the questions. Their answers were also more creative and easier to understand. Bananas are packed with potassium that keeps the brain, nerves, and heart in good health. The best part is that there is no cutting or slicing involved. All your child needs to do is peel and eat (Nolasco, 2014).

Spinach

As adults, we all have a fondness for spinach because we saw Popeye gain immense strength after consuming it straight from the tin. Spinach on its own is a crunchy, leafy vegetable that is rich in iron, folate, and vitamins A, C, and K. Not only is it good for muscle strength and bones but it is also excellent when it comes to improving mood and alertness. Spinach is also loaded with beta-carotene and lutein—two nutrients that have been linked with preventing dementia.

Chapter 7:

Healthy Eating for the Body

Eating healthy reduces the chances of disabilities and health conditions like osteoporosis, heart disease, and diabetes. The right foods can boost our mood, build immunity, as well as help with healthy sleeping patterns. Most healthy foods like fruits, vegetables, nuts, and seeds come packed with fiber, natural sugars, and vitamins that give our bodies an instant boost of energy when we need it the most. Eating fresh fruits and vegetables daily has also been linked with reduced risk of mental health conditions like depression, as they contain happiness-boosting nutrients that promote the production of dopamine in the cells. On the other hand, foods high in complex carbs and trans fats require long hours to be digested, leaving you feeling bloated, heavy, and lethargic.

Since the goal is to ensure that children consume only the most nutritious foods and drinks, in this final chapter, we look at how foods can boost energy, improve our stamina, improve immunity, and positively impact our mental and social health.

How Foods Boost Energy, Physical, and Mental Health

Weight gain and obesity are some of the most pressing concerns with parents these days. Unhealthy lunches, binge eating, and midnight snacking are practices that are linked with unwanted weight gain among children and teenagers. The first step to staying fit and healthy is attaining a normal weight. Heavy children give their bones extra work. The more pressure there is on their legs, the weaker and more brittle they become over time. If the goal is to help your child maintain a healthy weight, there are many foods like whole grains, lean meats, and leafy vegetables that can help. Having these in abundance can help maintain a healthy weight and prevent weight gain. Combine that with moderate-level exercise, and your child can easily shed off the extra pounds they gained over the holidays.

To understand how food can play a key role in the maintenance of healthy weight, researchers looked at three different diets and analyzed their effects. A low-fat, calorie-restricted diet might have proven effective, but as it turns out, it was Mediterranean diets with olive oil and nuts that proved the healthiest. Mediterranean diets include a balanced intake of fruits and vegetables that promote good immune health. They also improve blood pressure levels, fight inflammation, and improve insulin sensitivity. When the body sustains a healthy weight, there are fewer chances of bone-related injuries and conditions. Improved immunity means that the body has the power to fight off bacteria and viruses efficiently. Normal blood pressure levels mean fewer chances of developing cardiovascular disease (Widmer et al., 2015).

A healthy and well-rounded diet also benefits your child's psyche. They can learn to identify a hunger cue and differentiate it from a craving or trigger. They can know when to stop when they feel satisfied. They must know that they don't necessarily have to eat until they are full. This simple trick can keep their blood sugar levels and energy in check. When they eat to satisfy and enjoy different flavors and textures, they can amp up their mood. There is an emerging science that links your gut health with positive brain experiences, moods, and mental clarity. The right foods can make you feel more in control by boosting energy and improving your mood so that you can experience more positive feelings.

Students dealing with the pressures of good grades, college applications, and social interactions can prove to be a promising aspect.

Overall, the right nutrients work as a manual by telling the body how to function. Learning to think about food this way can help your child take note of their daily calorie intake, resist temptations, and not give in to their cravings. It can teach them how to differentiate between good and bad foods based on the reaction of their body to it.

Best Foods for a Stronger and Healthier Child

When you plant a garden, you want the best soil and fertilizers to put in. You ensure that your plants get the most sunlight and water. Imagine the results if you put in cheap quality soil and poor quality fertilizers. You forget to water the plants or plant them in a shaded area. What can you expect? You may still have a plant sprouting out of the ground, but it won't be well shaped and healthy looking.

In other words, giving your child the best nutrients and foods will yield the best results. They will have a healthy weight and be stronger, sharper, and happier than other children. A lot of the time, parents focus so much on what they should exclude from their child's diet that they forget about the more important aspect of it: What foods you should give to boost physical and mental health.

Below are some foods that should be on your "Must Give My Child List" because they guarantee instant energy, healthy body weight, improved gut, better immune health, and mental peace.

Fatty Fish

Fatty fish like tuna and salmon are rich sources of protein. They contain fatty acids, omega-3s, and vitamin

B, making them a healthy alternative to eating poultry or meat every day. Omega-3 fatty acids reduce inflammation which leads to fatigue—both physical and mental. It also contains healthy folate and vitamin B12 that help in the production of red blood cells. The greater the quantity of these cells in your body, the easier it is for iron to work better. Iron, also found in apples, is known to boost energy and ease fatigue.

Leafy Greens

Leafy vegetables like cabbage, spinach, parsley, mint, kale, and lettuce are all rich in antioxidants and carotenoids that enhance brain power and gut health. Leafy greens are easy to digest and are excess in vitamin A and B. Some vegetables like spinach, kale, cabbage and Brussels sprouts are also high in folic acids which are cell-building blocks.

Nuts and Seeds

A combination of nuts and seeds can serve as a healthy snack to munch on. They both are powerhouses for the brain and body. They are high in fatty acids that promote mental and physical health. Nuts are also high in vitamin E which is essential for children. Vitamin E has neuroprotective benefits, and it prevents cognitive decline in adults. Children who have a difficult time staying focused benefit by incorporating nuts like almonds, hazelnuts, sunflower seeds, and Brazil nuts into their diet.

Apples

Apples are the most commonly enjoyed fruit around the globe and for all the right reasons. For starters, there are over 25 different kinds of apples found in various parts of the world. Second, they are an excellent source of iron, fiber, and carbs. A medium-sized apple contains 2.4 grams of fiber, 13.8 grams of carbs, and 10.4 grams of simple sugars. The amount of fiber present in apples slows down the breakdown of sugar, promoting sustained energy release (Arnarson, 2019).

Yogurt

Yogurt is a great snack to fuel the body with stamina and energy. Its regular intake makes for excellent immunity and wellness. Yogurt contains probiotics that increase the number of healthy gut bacteria. It is easy to digest and can be consumed in many ways. Yogurt is made of simple sugars that are easy to break down; thus, there is an instant energy boost! As it is a type of dairy, it also comes packed with protein.

Strawberries

Nearly all kinds of berries have something special to offer. Like bananas, they are also instant energy boosting and fulfilling fruit. They are loaded with carbs, sugars, and fiber that boost energy levels. Strawberries also help with recovery and healing. They do so by fighting inflammation (Tardy et al., 2020). They are also ideal to consume when one feels lethargic and fatigued.

Like most fruits, they can be incorporated into many different recipes, salads, smoothies, and desserts.

Conclusion

We all know that healthy eating can transform our lives and help us live longer. We want the same for our children. We want to see them grow up stronger than ever. We want them to face everyday challenges actively and confidently. But where does healthy eating come in with all of this, and what do we mean by healthy eating?

In this book, we have tried to help parents come face-to-face with the challenges they face with a toddler or teenager and their unhealthy eating practices. From engaging in junk food to being a picky eater, we know the struggles parents face. However, this isn't a lost war. No matter how young or old your child is, there is always time to encourage healthy eating. By giving them a variety of healthy options to pick from, you can break their bad eating habits.

This book answers all your questions from debunking child nutrition myths to what foods are best for mental and physical health.

Remember: This transformation won't happen overnight. Your child won't wake up craving fruits and vegetables. This process takes time, patience, and encouragement on your part. You don't need to take control over what they eat: You need to help them steer their preferences from bad to good. You need to carve in the wisdom so that they know why eating a salad is better than a burger and fries.

With the tips and actionable steps discussed in this book, it shouldn't be hard. Hopefully, if you follow the ideas shared, you should have an amazing child willing to try on new and exciting healthy foods and recipes.

Thank you for giving this book a read. I hope you loved reading it as much as I enjoyed writing it. It would make me the happiest person on earth if you would take a moment to leave an honest review. All you have to do is visit the site where you purchased this book: It's that simple! The review doesn't have to be a full-fledged paragraph; a few words will do. Your few words will help others decide if this is what they should be reading as well. Thank you in advance, and best of luck with your parenting adventures. Every moment is a joyous one with a child.

References

7 foods for focus and concentration | heights. (2021, February 11). Www.yourheights.com. https://www.yourheights.com/blog/nutrition/foods-for-focus-and-concentration

7 popular kid nutrition myths debunked. (n.d.). Land O' Frost. Retrieved October 29, 2021, from https://www.landofrost.com/7-popular-kid-nutrition-myths-debunked/

8 myths about child nutrition that need to end today. (n.d.). Www.asknestle.in. Retrieved October 29, 2021, from https://www.asknestle.in/expert-advice/8-myths-about-child-nutrition-need-end-today

Arnarson, A. (2019, May 8). *Apples 101: Nutrition Facts and Health Benefits.* Healthline. https://www.healthline.com/nutrition/foods/apples

Bailey, C. (2018, April 27). *9 brain foods that will improve your focus and concentration.* A Life of Productivity.

https://alifeofproductivity.com/9-brain-foods-that-will-boost-your-ability-to-focus/

Benjamin, E. J., Muntner, P., Alonso, A., Bittencourt, M. S., Callaway, C. W., Carson, A. P., Chamberlain, A. M., Chang, A. R., Cheng, S., Das, S. R., Delling, F. N., Djousse, L., Elkind, M. S. V., Ferguson, J. F., Fornage, M., Jordan, L. C., Khan, S. S., Kissela, B. M., Knutson, K. L., & Kwan, T. W. (2019). Heart disease and stroke statistics—2019 update: A report from the american heart association. *Circulation, 139*(10). https://doi.org/10.1161/cir.0000000000000659

Bernstein, S. (2016, April 22). *Healthy eating: Nutrients kids need.* WebMD. https://www.webmd.com/parenting/features/4-nutrients-your-child-may-be-missing#1

Bilich, K. A. (2005, October 4). *9 must-eat nutrients for your child.* Parents; Parents. https://www.parents.com/kids/nutrition/healthy-eating/must-eat-nutrients/

Breymeyer, K. L., Lampe, J. W., McGregor, B. A., & Neuhouser, M. L. (2016). Subjective mood and energy levels of healthy weight and overweight/obese healthy adults on high-and low-glycemic load experimental diets. *Appetite, 107*, 253–259. https://doi.org/10.1016/j.appet.2016.08.008

CDC. (2019). *Childhood nutrition facts.* Centers for Disease Control and Prevention. https://www.cdc.gov/healthyschools/nutrition/facts.htm

Cepeda, A. M., Thawer, S., Boyle, R. J., Villalba, S., Jaller, R., Tapias, E., Segura, A. M., Villegas, R., & Garcia-Larsen, V. (2017). Diet and respiratory health in children from 11 latin american countries: Evidence from ISAAC phase III. *Lung, 195*(6), 683–692. https://doi.org/10.1007/s00408-017-0044-z

Clifford, T., Howatson, G., West, D., & Stevenson, E. (2015). The potential benefits of red beetroot supplementation in health and disease. *Nutrients, 7*(4), 2801–2822. https://doi.org/10.3390/nu7042801

Conner, T. S., Brookie, K. L., Richardson, A. C., & Polak, M. A. (2015). On carrots and curiosity: Eating fruit and vegetables is associated with greater flourishing in daily life. *British Journal of Health Psychology, 20*(2), 413–427. https://doi.org/10.1111/bjhp.12113

Crichton-Stuart, C. (2020, December 10). *The top 10 benefits of eating healthy*. Www.medicalnewstoday.com. https://www.medicalnewstoday.com/articles/322268

Dominguez, L. J., & Barbagallo, M. (2018). Nutritional prevention of cognitive decline and dementia. *Acta Bio Medica: Atenei Parmensis*, *89*(2), 276.

Eating disorders and adolescents. (2012). Vic.gov.au. https://www.betterhealth.vic.gov.au/health/healthyliving/eating-disorders-adolescents

Eating disorders in children and adolescents. (2020, December 21). Hopkinsallchildrens.org; Johns Hopkins All Children's Hospital. https://www.hopkinsallchildrens.org/ACH-News/General-News/Eating-Disorders-in-Children-and-Adolescents

Eating your way to focus and concentration. (2017, October 4). Psychology Compass. https://psychologycompass.com/blog/eating-your-way-to-focus-and-concentration/

Field, L. (2018, March 21). *5 nutrition myths about kids & food*. Nurture Life. https://www.nurturelife.com/blog/5-kid-food-myths-debunked/

Friedman, R. (2014, October 17). *What you eat affects your productivity*. Harvard Business Review. https://hbr.org/2014/10/what-you-eat-affects-your-productivity

Hatter, K. (2018, December 5). *The benefits of eating healthy foods as a child.* Hello Motherhood. https://www.hellomotherhood.com/the-benefits-of-eating-healthy-foods-as-a-child-5762623.html

Health benefits of eating well. (2020, April 30). Nhsinform.scot. https://www.nhsinform.scot/healthy-living/food-and-nutrition/eating-well/health-benefits-of-eating-well

How your eating habits affect your health & how to change them. (2019, March 14). Advanced Body Scan. https://advancedbodyscan.com/how-your-eating-habits-affect-your-health-how-to-change-them/

Hoyland, A., Dye, L., & Lawton, C. L. (2009). A systematic review of the effect of breakfast on the cognitive performance of children and adolescents. *Nutrition Research Reviews*, *22*(2), 220–243. https://doi.org/10.1017/s0954422409990175

Indian parenting website, kids website in india, activities & events for children in india. (2017, August 7). Kidsstoppress. https://www.kidsstoppress.com/details/myths-and-facts-when-it-comes-to-complete-nutrition-of-your-child/13521

Kam, K. (2007, September 10). *Eating disorders in children and teens.* WebMD; WebMD. https://www.webmd.com/mental-health/eating-disorders/features/eating-disorders-children-teens

Malik, V. (2019, September 4). *National nutrition week 2019: Common myths about kids' nutrition debunked.* Only My Health. https://www.onlymyhealth.com/5-common-diet-myths-that-can-hamper-your-child-s-health-1567601778

Maxwell, L. (2012, September 14). *Six nutrition myths debunked.* On the Pulse. https://pulse.seattlechildrens.org/six-nutrition-myths-debunked/

Mclaughlin, A. (2008). *How does eating healthy affect your physical, mental & social health?* Sfgate.com. https://healthyeating.sfgate.com/eating-healthy-affect-physical-mental-social-health-6972.html

MLaughlin, A. (2012). *The benefits of eating healthy foods as a child.* Sfgate.com. https://healthyeating.sfgate.com/benefits-eating-healthy-foods-child-4302.html

Mohajeri, M. H., Wittwer, J., Vargas, K., Hogan, E., Holmes, A., Rogers, P. J., Goralczyk, R., & Gibson, E. L. (2015). Chronic treatment with a tryptophan-rich protein hydrolysate improves emotional processing, mental energy levels and reaction time in middle-aged women. *The British Journal of Nutrition, 113*(2), 350–365. https://doi.org/10.1017/S0007114514003754

Nolasco, S. (2014, July 21). *10 foods that boost concentration.* Health.com. https://www.health.com/food/10-foods-that-boost-concentration

Physical health - food. (2019, July 11). Www.headtohealth.gov.au. https://www.headtohealth.gov.au/meaningful-life/physical-health/food

Rampersaud, G. C., Pereira, M. A., Girard, B. L., Adams, J., & Metzl, J. D. (2005). Breakfast habits, nutritional status, body weight, and academic performance in children and adolescents. *Journal of the American Dietetic Association*, *105*(5), 743–760. https://doi.org/10.1016/j.jada.2005.02.007

Revelant, J. (2018, December 11). *6 real reasons parents don't feed their kids healthy food.* Julie Revelant | Raise Healthy Kids Who Crave Healthy Food. https://www.julierevelant.com/6-real-reasons-parents-dont-feed-their-kids-healthy-food/

Richardson, M. (2019, February 1). *How Much Energy Does the Brain Use?* BrainFacts.org. https://www.brainfacts.org/brain-anatomy-and-function/anatomy/2019/how-much-energy-does-the-brain-use-020119

Ruth, A. (2019, January 23). *How nutrition can affect your focus and productivity throughout the day.* Calendar. https://www.calendar.com/blog/focus-and-productivity/

Santiago-Rodríguez, E., Estrada-Zaldívar, B., & Zaldívar-Uribe, E. (2018). Effects of dark chocolate intake on brain electrical oscillations in healthy people. *Foods*, *7*(11), 187. https://doi.org/10.3390/foods7110187

Segal, J., & Robinson, L. (2021, August). *Healthy food for kids.* Https://Www.helpguide.org.

https://www.helpguide.org/articles/healthy-eating/healthy-food-for-kids.htm#

Semeco, A. (2017, December 4). *27 foods that can give you more energy*. Healthline; Healthline Media. https://www.healthline.com/nutrition/energy-boosting-foods

Shan, Z., Li, Y., Baden, M. Y., Bhupathiraju, S. N., Wang, D. D., Sun, Q., Rexrode, K. M., Rimm, E. B., Qi, L., Willett, W. C., Manson, J. E., Qi, Q., & Hu, F. B. (2020). Association between healthy eating patterns and risk of cardiovascular disease. *JAMA Internal Medicine, 180*(8), 1090. https://doi.org/10.1001/jamainternmed.2020.2176

Statista. (2020). *Number of McDonald's restaurants in North America from 2012 to 2020, by country*. Statista. https://www.statista.com/statistics/256040/mcdonalds-restaurants-in-north-america/

Taras, H. (2005). Nutrition and student performance at school. *Journal of School Health*, *75*(6), 199–213. https://doi.org/10.1111/j.1746-1561.2005.00025.x

Tardy, A.-L., Pouteau, E., Marquez, D., Yilmaz, C., & Scholey, A. (2020). Vitamins and minerals for energy, fatigue and cognition: A narrative review of the biochemical and clinical evidence. *Nutrients*, *12*(1), 228. https://doi.org/10.3390/nu12010228

Types of eating disorders in children & adolescents. (2019). Nyulangone.org. https://nyulangone.org/conditions/eating-disorders-in-children-adolescents/types

U.S. Department of Health and Human Services; U.S. Department of Agriculture (2015). 2015–2020 Dietary Guidelines for Americans. 8th Edition. Available at http://health.gov/dietaryguidelines/2015/guidelines/

Widmer, R. J., Flammer, A. J., Lerman, L. O., & Lerman, A. (2015). The mediterranean diet, its components, and cardiovascular disease. *The American Journal of Medicine*, *128*(3), 229–238. https://doi.org/10.1016/j.amjmed.2014.10.014

www.ingramcontent.com/pod-product-compliance
Lightning Source LLC
LaVergne TN
LVHW051017080826
845145LV00009B/2675

* 9 7 8 1 9 5 6 0 1 8 2 3 3 *